Locum Pharmacy

Locum Pharmacy

A survival guide

Pamela Mason

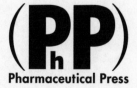

Pharmaceutical Press

Published by the Pharmaceutical Press
1 Lambeth High Street, London SE1 7JN

First edition 1998

© 1998 Pharmaceutical Press

Text design by Barker/Hilsdon
Typeset by Photoprint, Torquay, Devon
Printed in Great Britain by TJ International, Padstow, Cornwall

ISBN 0 85369 397 8

A catalogue record for this book is available from the British Library

Contents

Preface

'My grandmother died yesterday. The funeral is on Friday. Can you cover for me?' If you become a locum pharmacist, you will probably get used to receiving telephone calls like this. Indeed, locums are often organised at very short notice, and provided you apply yourself efficiently, professionally and productively, you will rapidly become sought after. You will always be asked back and you will, at least in the current community pharmacy climate, never be short of work.

Locums are in great demand, for several reasons. First, many pharmacy multiples have difficulty in filling their permanent pharmacist posts. Second, the fact that many community pharmacies open increasingly long hours means that two or more pharmacists are needed to cover the working week. Third, some pharmacists are involved in additional pharmacy services (e.g. advising general practitioners on prescribing, medication review in nursing/residential homes, domiciliary visits etc.) or perhaps in continuing education activities which may take them away from the pharmacy and result in the need for a locum. Quite simply, if you are a good locum, your telephone will probably never stop ringing.

But if you want to do locums and you have not got much experience, where do you start? What factors do you need to consider? How do you obtain work? What questions should you ask before accepting a locum booking? And what about your first day in an unfamiliar pharmacy – how do you cope? What should you watch out for? What will be expected of you? What personal financial records should you keep and how do you pay your income tax? Should you have an accountant? Should you consider professional indemnity insurance? What about a pension and life assurance?

The aim of this book is to provide a unique, handy guide to working as a locum in community pharmacy, particularly if you are new to locuming, working in a community pharmacy or both. My own experience as a locum pharmacist has convinced me of the need for this book, and much of its content has been drawn from my own work as a locum or the experience of colleagues and friends.

Pamela Mason
London
April, 1998

1

Introduction

You might choose to do locums for all sorts of reasons. Some pharmacists make locums their full-time occupation, but some choose to do locums at weekends while working in another branch of the profession during the week. For pharmacists who work, say, in academia, industry or as consultants, doing the odd locum can be a useful way of staying in touch. Pharmacists who are parents often find the flexibility of locuming and the facility to work part time useful while the children are young. Newly qualifieds frequently value the experience of working in different pharmacies for a while.

WHO CAN DO LOCUMS?

To do locums in Great Britain, you must be registered as a pharmacist with the Royal Pharmaceutical Society of Great Britain (RPSGB). If you have qualified as a pharmacist in another country, you will need to fulfil various requirements prior to registration in the UK. If your country is a member of the European Union and you can provide evidence that your qualifications and training fulfil the current EU Directive, you will be able to register and work as a pharmacist in Great Britain almost straight away. If you are registered in Australia or New Zealand – countries with which the RPSGB has a reciprocal agreement – again, little formality is involved, and following an interview and a month's experience in a British pharmacy, you will be free to work on your own account.

If you come from a country which is neither a member of the EU nor has a reciprocal agreement with the RPSGB, you may need to do further training and you will be required to complete a pre-registration year and pass a registration examination. This whole process could take about two years.

WHAT DOES BEING A LOCUM INVOLVE?

The term locum is short for 'locum tenens', which, translated literally, means 'holding the place'. Not by any means an easy option, being a locum means that you have all the responsibilities of a manager or proprietor without necessarily being familiar with the pharmacy.

Professional obligations

As a locum, your professional obligations are the same as those of any other pharmacist and you can find details of these in *Medicines, Ethics and Practice – A guide for pharmacists* (published by the Royal Pharmaceutical Society of Great Britain). However, in particular you must:

○ Be aware of the Code of Ethics and the Guide to Good Dispensing.

○ Provide all the necessary information to patients on the safe use and administration of medicines – both over the counter and prescribed medicines.

○ Supervise all sales of pharmacy (P) medicines; when the pharmacist is absent, no P medicines must be sold.

○ Give relevant and up-to-date advice on all matters concerning health and medication and refer patients to their general practitioner when appropriate.

○ Be available to intervene in discussions at the medicines counter on any aspect of medication or health education.

Specific tasks

In addition to fulfilling your professional obligations, working in a pharmacy involves many specific tasks. What exactly is required of you as a locum will vary from pharmacy to pharmacy and may depend on the experience and training of the staff as well as the working practices of the manager or proprietor. As a guide, however, each day you may be expected to:

○ Endorse, count, record and file prescriptions.

○ Order dispensary and counter items and transmit orders to wholesalers and manufacturers.

○ Complete an end-of-day backup on the computer.

○ Cash up and bank the takings.

○ Pay staff wages.

○ Lock up the pharmacy and set the burglar alarm.

○ Deliver prescriptions to patients' homes and nursing and residential homes.

At the end of the week you may be required to:

○ Add up prescription numbers – if you are working for a pharmacy multiple, this might include sending prescription statistics to the company's head office.

○   Display rota/bank holiday signs.

At the end of the month you may be required to:

○   Complete end-of-month paperwork for prescriptions and send prescriptions to the pricing bureau.

○   Change sales promotions, particularly if you are working for a multiple.

WHAT ARE THE ADVANTAGES?

Working as a locum offers several advantages, and which of the following features you would value the most will obviously depend on your personal circumstances. Thus:

○   You are largely your own boss.

○   You can work when and where you like.

○   You can, to some extent, control what you earn.

○   You can work as many or as few hours as you want.

○   You can gain experience and skills in many different types of pharmacy.

○   You can find out what type of pharmacy you most enjoy working in before committing yourself to a permanent position.

○   You can normally leave the pharmacy, forget the day's work and not go home to a pile of paperwork.

○   The pharmacy staff generally do not have time to get fed up with you, nor you with them!

WHAT ARE THE DISADVANTAGES?

Just like any other way of practising your profession and earning a living, locuming has disadvantages too, and you may wish to consider these, particularly if you are thinking about leaving a permanent job and locuming full time. Thus:

○ Your hours could fluctuate enormously – anything from 9 until 5.30 p.m. to 8 until 10 p.m. – and this does not just include the pharmacy opening hours. You may, for example, find yourself delivering medicines to patients at home and to residential and nursing homes after the pharmacy has closed. Think about the impact on your social and family life.

○ You need to adapt to different surroundings and work within other people's systems – you will probably need to get to know at least half a dozen computer systems, as well as several types of cash register and burglar alarms.

○ You will rarely have the opportunity to see things through, since you may work in a different place every day.

○ Travelling and finding a new place, particularly if you are working in a different place each week, can be exhausting.

○ You may be free to work when there is none available, although currently this is quite rare, at least in many areas of the UK. What is more likely is that, having booked up your week, you may be wanted several times over.

○ Your income is not guaranteed and could fluctuate.

○ You need to provide for your own pension, holiday pay, sick pay and income tax.

IS IT FOR YOU?

Think carefully about the pros and cons. Locuming can be a great deal of fun, you will probably make a great number of friends and may relish the freedom and flexibility. Depending on your circumstances and personality, however, you might find the lack of routine and fluctuating income more than you can handle. Only you can decide what you can live with.

2

Getting started

If you decide you want to do locums, there are several things, some professional, some personal and some practical, which you need to think about before you start. For example, how long is it since you worked in a pharmacy? Do you want to work locally or are you prepared to travel? Do you have access to a car? What is your local public transport like? Are you planning to work as a locum full time or part time? Perhaps you work in another branch of pharmacy during the week and you intend to locum just at weekends. Perhaps you have had a career break and you want to ease yourself back into pharmacy by doing locums.

RETURN TO PRACTICE

If you have not worked as a pharmacist for a while, or even if you work regularly in another branch of the profession, working in a community pharmacy can be quite daunting. Consider participating in one of the Centre for Pharmacy Postgraduate Education's Return to Practice workshops or ordering their Return to Practice distance learning materials. The workshop is structured to run over a period of one week or a weekend, or you can choose to do it on a daily basis on five separate days. The distance learning material is in the form of an interactive video and accompanying workbook. Both, of course, are free of charge.

The National Pharmaceutical Association runs courses on the Drug Tariff and truss fitting. These are open to NPA members only, but you should be able to access one by virtue of working in a member's pharmacy.

FEES

If you are returning to pharmacy practice after a break, you may only be paying a reduced registration fee to the Royal Pharmaceutical Society. Remember that if your locum work results in you exceeding a total of 13 weeks' employment in a year, you must pay the full registration fee. All paid employment, as a pharmacist or otherwise, must be included.

TELEPHONE

At the very least, you will need a telephone answering machine at home. But you may also want to consider having a mobile phone. Mobile phones are not that expensive to run, particularly if you use them mainly for incoming calls, and it does, of course, mean that prospective clients can get hold of you immediately. By the time you get home at night and respond to your answerphone messages, any work may already have gone to someone who can be contacted immediately.

PRINTED STATIONERY

Business cards are a must. Include your qualifications as well as your contact details (address; telephone, facsimile and mobile numbers; and e-mail, whichever you have). A business card is a useful advertisement. Leaving one at every pharmacy you work often generates a surprising amount of business. You may also want to consider headed notepaper. This is useful if you want to advertise your services by writing round to local pharmacies. I sometimes use it for writing out receipts for locum fees.

TRANSPORT

If you own or have the use of a car, transport will be no problem, and you can accept work anywhere. But if you have to rely solely on public transport, you may have to pick and choose where you work. Of course, if you plan only to work locally, a bike or a decent pair of shoes will be all you need!

DIARY

A comprehensive diary is another must. You might even consider keeping two – a pocket diary to carry about with you and a desk diary, or perhaps a calendar, next to the phone at home. But whatever you do, always write down dates then and there. And if you do decide to maintain two diaries, remember to cross refer them – every day, if possible. Writing down dates on scraps of paper and backs of envelopes, which have the habit of floating away into drawers and waste paper bins, is not a good idea. You cannot afford to get a reputation for double booking and losing the names and addresses of pharmacies in which you have agreed to work.

In your diary, make sure you make a note (at least) of the following:

○ The name, address and telephone number of the pharmacy.

○   The date(s) and hours you have agreed to work.

○   Fee or rate of pay and travel expenses.

As time goes on, you may also choose to use your diary for making notes about individual pharmacies, including perhaps the different computer systems. For example, I use the back of my diary to record basic instructions for producing labels, owings slips and ordering on each of the computer systems I work with. This can be a useful memory jogger and can save a lot of time if you cannot find the computer instructions manual in the pharmacy.

Your diary can also be useful for keeping a note of business telephone numbers, for example those of pharmacies and agencies for whom you work regularly, other local pharmacies, other locum pharmacists, local doctors and local health authorities, frequently used wholesalers and suppliers, the Royal Pharmaceutical Society, the National Pharmaceutical Association and the Pharmaceutical Services Negotiating Committee.

FILING

You might want to consider setting up a filing system for your locum work. This could include business correspondence and records of income and expenses, contact names and addresses as well as reference and resource materials.

KEEPING UP TO DATE

This, of course, is vital wherever you work, but you may have to work a bit harder at it if you are self-employed. You might find the following suggestions helpful:

○ Read your *Pharmaceutical Journal* regularly. Get used to looking particularly at the news, clinical and new products pages. When you are working in a pharmacy, keep an eye out for the *Chemist & Druggist* (normally delivered on Fridays) and other pharmacy magazines.

○ Join the NPA as a 'publications' subscriber. (Locum pharmacists will only be accepted as subscribers if all the pharmacies they work in are NPA members. This covers nearly all community pharmacies in the UK except those belonging to Boots.) Publications subscription entitles you to all the literature and leaflets sent out by the association to its members, e.g. the *NPA Supplement*, the *NPA Guide to the Drug Tariff*, and revised and new information leaflets such as vaccine requirements for travelling abroad and malaria prophylaxis. Being a publications subscriber also entitles you to take advantage of NPA personal services such as NPA travel, private healthcare and car purchase and finance, but it does not give access to other member services, such as the information department or advice on legal, financial, taxation or employment matters. While working in an NPA member's pharmacy, you can, of course, use the NPA's information department by virtue of the member's subscription.

○ Make sure you are on the mailing list of one of the Centres for Pharmacy Postgraduate Education – in England, Scotland or Wales, depending where you live. They regularly send out details of distance learning packs for self study and workshops taking place in your geographical area.

○ Read the *MeReC Bulletin* regularly. You will receive this with your *Pharmaceutical Journal*.

○ Consider taking out a subscription to the *Drug & Therapeutics Bulletin*. This will help you to keep up to date on new drugs and therapeutic issues. The cost of a year's subscription is £30.75 from the NPA.

○   Attend conferences, exhibitions and trade shows as often as you can.

○   Buy or send for relevant reports, leaflets, bulletins, news-letters and fact sheets. You will often find information about these in the *Pharmaceutical Journal*.

○   Make contact with your local drug information and post-graduate medical centres. They will normally do searches and provide with you with up-to-date articles on, for example, disease management and new drug treatments.

○   Make use of the Internet, if you have access to it.

3

Getting work

Once you have decided to work as a locum, you need to get yourself known. You might find some or all of the following methods useful:

○ Visit your local pharmacies, chat to the owners, tell them about your experience and leave a business card.

○ Write to local pharmacies and enclose a copy of your curriculum vitae. If you include pharmacy multiples on your list, try to find out who in the company co-ordinates locums and write to these people.

○ Look through your local Yellow Pages to identify other pharmacies which you have not contacted.

○ Enrol with locum agencies. You will find their names and telephone numbers in the advertisement section of the *Pharmaceutical Journal* (see also Appendix 2). Note that many agencies focus on particular parts of the country, so find out which areas are covered.

○ Look in the *Pharmaceutical Journal* and *Chemist & Druggist* for locum advertisements.

○ Put a personal advertisement in the *Pharmaceutical Journal*. You will find the cost of doing this at the top of the first page in the classified section of the journal.

○ Look for work on the Internet. Locums are advertised on the *Chemist & Druggist's* web site (http://www.dotpharmacy. co.uk). You can also register your availability on the Internet.

○   Circulate at local CPPE workshops and RPSGB and NPA branch meetings.

○   Contact your local RPSGB or NPA branch secretary who may keep lists of locums for circulation to local pharmacies. Some local wholesalers also keep such lists.

○   Tell any pharmacy sales representatives you meet that you are looking for work; they may pass your name on to other pharmacies on their travels.

CONSIDERING JOB OFFERS

Consider offers of work carefully, particularly if you have had a career break or you are new to community pharmacy. A challenge is a challenge, but do not take on work which is well beyond your capability and experience. Try and find out how busy the pharmacy is, both with prescriptions and over-the-counter work, before you accept an offer of work there. If you have not dispensed a prescription for five years, or even six months, and take an offer of work in a pharmacy doing over 200 items a day, you will be in for a nasty shock and by the end of the day you may never want to see the inside of a pharmacy again. If the dispensary is busy, find out if there is a technician to help you.

If in doubt, go and look at the pharmacy and ask to be shown round and meet the staff. Does the pharmacy look clean and tidy? Are the storage systems and equipment adequate? If you are relatively new to community pharmacy, it can be a nightmare working in one which is untidy and badly organised.

Indeed, if you are really out of practice, the best thing is to contact one of your local pharmacies and see if you can work for a couple of mornings with the owner, unpaid, so that you can begin to find your feet again.

LOCUM AGREEMENT FORMS

If you agree to work in a pharmacy where you have not worked before, you and the owner should fill in and sign a locum agreement form. Many pharmacies keep these forms in stock, but you can obtain them for yourself from the NPA. Once filled in, the form will remain in force for any subsequent bookings you make at that pharmacy, or if the agreement is with a pharmacy multiple, the completed form covers you for working in any branch belonging to that company. This form will also be recognised by the Inland Revenue as evidence of your self-employed status for tax purposes (see Chapter 9).

MAKING A BOOKING

The time when you make a booking may be the only time you speak to the owner or manager of the pharmacy. At this point, it is therefore crucial that you are well organised with your questions ready and your diary at hand to write down all the relevant details. I always find it useful to have a map handy to check roughly where the pharmacy is and how far it is to travel.

You might want to develop your own checklist of questions to ask the regular pharmacist, but in particular make sure that you:

○   Check booking dates.

○   Write down the telephone number of the pharmacy and an emergency contact number for the owner or regular manager/ pharmacist.

○   Check the name and full address of the pharmacy. Check that there are not two roads of the same or similar name in the town, and check that there are not two towns of the same name in the same district. The owner or agency may send you a map, if you ask. But make absolutely certain where you are supposed to go!

○   Find out the hours you are expected to work. This can often be later than the time the pharmacy closes, particularly if you have to make deliveries. In addition you may be expected to do a rota (including a Sunday rota). There is nothing worse than having made arrangements to go out for the evening or having told your childminder that you will be back at 6 p.m., only to discover that the shop you are working in is on rota until 7 p.m.

It is also helpful to find out:

○   What the local rush hour traffic is like in the morning.

○   If there are car parking facilities next to the pharmacy or where the best place to park is.

○   Which computer system is used in the pharmacy.

○   How many support staff you will be working with and what their relative levels of experience, training and responsibilities are. In particular find out if dispensary staff know how to use the computer and what hours the staff work.

○   What arrangements are made for lunch-times. Does the pharmacy close or not? If, as is increasingly the case, the pharmacy remains open at lunch-time, ask what arrangements are usually made for pharmacy cover at lunch-times. If you are expected to stay on the premises, make sure you are going to be paid for doing so.

○   If there are any registered drug addicts and how many.

○   If the pharmacy services nursing/residential homes, how many and on which days of the week.

○   If you are expected to deliver to nursing/residential homes or hospices or to deliver oxygen.

○   If the pharmacy offers any other extra services (e.g. needle exchange schemes) and what they are.

○   If you are expected to cash up and bank the takings; if so, check that the owner or manager will leave a note regarding all the banking details.

○   What arrangements are made for locking up, setting the burglar alarm and/or holding the keys to the pharmacy.

○   What professional indemnity insurance is provided. Ask if the pharmacy belongs to the NPA. Double check by asking for the NPA membership number, and if in doubt, check its validity with the NPA. (The locum agencies tend to do this for you.) You might also wish to consider having your own professional indemnity cover (see Chapter 10).

Some pharmacies have a folder or book which gives details of procedures for locums, names and telephone numbers of local doctors, nursing and residential homes and also contact numbers for various types of emergencies (e.g. broken glass, failure of burglar alarm etc.).

NEGOTIATING FEES

Talking about money can be a difficult issue. Work for an agency or a pharmacy multiple and the rates are fixed so you do not have to worry. But if you work for independents, you will have to negotiate your own fee.

When thinking about the rate you want to charge, it is worthwhile considering the following points:

○   If you are too greedy, it is not likely that you will be asked again.

○   Do not sell yourself too cheap. Not only does this undervalue your professional worth, but it will also annoy other locums.

○   As guidance, you can refer to the rates paid by agencies and multiples and ask your locum friends what they charge.

○   Locum rates of pay tend to vary from area to area. This depends on market forces to some extent.

○   If you plan to work full time as a locum, calculate your rates based on a reasonable year's salary, including time off for holidays.

○   Do you want to charge on a daily or an hourly basis?

○   How much do you want to charge for working rotas, late evenings, Sundays and bank holidays?

Remember also to check when and how you will be paid. At one time – and this may still happen in some pharmacies – you took your money out of the till and left a receipt for the owner. However, most proprietors now pay by cheque and will leave one for you on the day you work. If you work for a multiple, you often have to fill in a form with the number of hours and days you have worked, send it to the company's head office and wait for the cheque to be posted to you. Such forms often require you to provide details of your tax district and national insurance number, so always have this information with you.

It is a good idea to keep records to check that you receive all your payments. If you have not been paid within four to six weeks, phone up the proprietor or company head office and ask if there are any queries over your payment. If payment still has not arrived within a few weeks, write and refer to your earlier phone call. Threatening legal action is the next step, but check out the appropriate procedure with your accountant or solicitor before doing this.

EXPENSES

Remember to ask about travel and accommodation expenses, unless the pharmacy is so near that you plan to walk or cycle.

Car

Car and motorbike expenses are usually paid by the mile. As a guide, if you want to fix your own car expenses, ring the AA or the RAC and ask them to provide you with figures for your make of vehicle. They will provide you with two sets of figures, one to cover running costs (e.g. petrol, tyres etc.) and one which covers running costs plus insurance, road tax etc. For example, for a car with a 1.8-litre engine capacity, the all inclusive figure works out at about 42 p/mile and for one with a 1.4-litre engine capacity, 33 p/mile. However, not everyone will be willing to pay these rates. Try checking with friends who have jobs which pay them travelling expenses, and find out what a reasonable rate would be.

If you work for a locum agency or multiple, expenses are often fixed in stone. Different companies make different arrangements. Some companies pay so much a mile for the first, say, 100 miles and nothing after that. Others pay nothing for the first, say, 20 miles and then pay so much a mile for the rest.

Public transport

If you plan to use public transport, you could ask for complete reimbursement of train, bus, tube or air fares. Get receipts for these, or at least keep your used tickets to pass on to your clients for their records.

Accommodation

Most locums travel to and from home each day, but sometimes you may want to accept a booking which takes you away overnight. Agree with the owner or manager beforehand what the cost of a reasonable night's accommodation would be in that particular area. They may arrange a hotel room for you.

A BOOKING IS A CONTRACT

Remember that when you have made a booking, either orally or in writing, you and the proprietor have made a binding contract. If having made a booking, you find that you are unavailable, you must get in touch with the proprietor immediately. If you have a good reason – bereavement or illness, for example – the proprietor will generally be sympathetic and willing to sort out the problem.

However, it is, in theory, your responsibility to find a replacement locum. So always keep other locums' phone numbers in your diary. If you fail to turn up or cannot provide a substitute, you could be sued for loss of profits if the pharmacy has to close. Conversely, if a proprietor cancels a booking at short notice and you are unable to find another place of work, you could sue the owner and take them to the small claims court. However, provided this does not happen regularly with one pharmacy, think carefully before taking another pharmacist to court.

4

At the pharmacy

This chapter deals with essential items to take with you to the pharmacy, and what to do when you arrive there for the first time.

WHAT TO TAKE WITH YOU

Your certificate

Always remember to take your certificate. By law, this must be displayed in the pharmacy in which you are working. If you have one of the older style large certificates, which are thoroughly inconvenient to carry, particularly on the bus, you can send it back to the RPSGB and ask for it to be replaced by an A4-sized one. This will generally take about four to six weeks, so you will be without your certificate during that time. If an RPSGB inspector comes into the pharmacy and your certificate is being replaced, an explanation to this effect should be acceptable.

Other items you may want to consider taking with you include:

○ A map.

○ Your diary, pens, a pair of scissors and a notebook.

○ Reference sources, e.g. the *BNF*; the RPSGB's *Medicines Ethics and Practice*; the *NPA Guide to the Drug Tariff*; one of the over-the-counter medicines guides (e.g. the *PAGB OTC*

Guide or the *Chemist & Druggist OTC Guide*); the current *Pharmaceutical Journal* and a current first aid manual; the NPA's leaflets on malaria prophylaxis, vaccination for travelling abroad and regulations for the supply and possession of Controlled Drugs.

○ An overall (although few community pharmacists now wear these).

GETTING THERE

Arrive in good time (i.e. about 10 minutes early). No matter how early you have to get up, allow plenty of time for travelling, particularly if the weather is bad. Even rain can considerably increase your journey time. If you are working at a pharmacy you have not worked in before, study a local map carefully to get a good idea of where you are going. Allow time for walking to and from the railway station, negotiating one-way streets and finding a place to park. Always carry plenty of change in case you have to use a 'pay and display' car park. In some parts of the country these can be expensive, and you may need several pounds' worth of change.

SETTLING IN

Arrive at the pharmacy looking smart and cheerful. No one wants to work with a miserable pharmacist! Introduce yourself to the staff and try to make them feel at ease. Remember that they will often feel uneasy about working with someone new. Find out where the regular pharmacist has gone on holiday – you will probably be asked this several times during the first two hours. Take time to look round the dispensary and the counter area.

THE DISPENSARY

Familiarise yourself, before you get busy, with the layout of the dispensary, particularly if there is no dispensing technician. Most dispensary items will generally be quite easy to find – they are usually stored alphabetically – but in particular, look (or ask a member of staff) for:

○ Items which may be kept separately from the rest (e.g. contraceptives, co-proxamol tablets, salbutamol inhalers, diabetic test kits, dressings, hosiery, injections, eye/ear drops, pessaries and suppositories).

○ Generic products, which are sometimes stored separately from branded products.

○ Fast moving items, which may be kept on a special shelf.

○ The refrigerator.

○ The Controlled Drugs cupboard and key. Remember that the CD key should be in your personal possession all the time the pharmacy is open.

○ The private prescriptions book and CD register.

○ Bags, bottles, ointment jars, spatulas, tape measure, spare dispensary stock and spare computer labels.

○   Dispensing balances and weights.

○   Fire extinguishers.

If you do not look for these items, you can be sure that when you need them, the only person in the pharmacy to know where they are will have gone out to lunch.

In addition, look out for letters and memos from local health authorities. They often send information to pharmacies about prescription forgeries in the area and many owners pin these letters on a notice board or above the dispensary bench.

SYSTEMS

Check what time orders arrive and when you should send orders to the wholesaler, including the deadlines for this (see also Chapter 7). Look at the computer (see also Chapter 6), and if it is a system with which you are not familiar, produce a test label using your own name. You can normally do this while bypassing the patient medication record system.

Try to find out early in the day how the pharmacy deals with medication which is owed to patients. Some pharmacies use computer generated slips, some handwritten slips, others just use word of mouth. If owings are recorded on the computer, make sure you find out how to cancel them.

If the pharmacy deals with addicts, check how many will require a supply of medicine that day. Ask about the system the pharmacy uses for servicing any nursing homes. For example, does a member of staff go round to the surgery to collect the prescriptions, or does the receptionist bring them round? Does the nursing home manager phone items through? And when and how are the medicines delivered?

If you are going to be at that pharmacy for more than a couple of days, get to know the local GP surgeries. Introduce yourself to the receptionists and let then know how long you are going to be there.

THE MEDICINES SALES AREA

Look on the medicines counter and see what products are stocked. There is nothing worse than recommending a specific cough mixture to a customer and finding out the pharmacy does not keep it in stock. Ask to be shown how the till works and what systems are used for taking in prescriptions and selling medicines.

If you are new to community pharmacy, you may be unfamiliar with over-the-counter medicines. The best way round this is to spend time on the medicines counter, familiarising yourself with products, their indications, contraindications and interactions with other medication. Obtain one of the OTC guides from either the Proprietary Association of Great Britain or the *Chemist & Druggist* (see Appendix 1 for further reference sources on OTC medicines and responding to symptoms).

Check the level of training and experience of the staff. All medicines counter staff must be trained on a course accredited by the RPSGB. Check what arrangements are made for the sales of pharmacy (P) medicines. Remember that P medicines should not be sold without the supervision of a pharmacist, so check how the staff will let you know that a customer wants to buy such a medicine. If you are unhappy with the pharmacy's system, do not be afraid to say so, and tell the staff exactly how you would like to deal with sales of medicines.

Ask if the pharmacy has a protocol and how the staff use it. If you consider the practice inadequate, again explain to them how you would like them to change it and why. It is up to you to lay down rules if there are none. In particular, highlight the types of request and products which you would like referring to yourself. This is particularly important with medicines which have only recently become available without prescription or those which are known to be subject to abuse.

If you leave the premises at lunch-time or any other time, make sure that the staff know not to sell pharmacy medicines. Also, make sure that a card informing customers of this is in a prominent place on the counter. It is vital that you inform the staff; if you do not do this, you will be liable should there be a prosecution (e.g. for the unsupervised sale of a P medicine).

WORKING WITH THE PHARMACY STAFF

Treat the pharmacy staff with courtesy and respect and they will be your allies. Many of them may have known the area for a lot longer than you have. They may have worked in the pharmacy for several years and be a mine of information. In my experience, most are kind and friendly, offering you cups of tea and coffee and running out to the baker's for your lunch if you want them to. Return these kindnesses whenever you can. Take your turn making the tea, and remember that treating them to cakes or biscuits on a Saturday afternoon never goes amiss! But if you get on the wrong side of the staff, you can pay for it in all sorts of ways.

In addition:

○ Try to follow the systems which normally operate in the pharmacy, unless you consider the working practices to be unprofessional or dangerous. You are used to working in different pharmacies with a variety of systems, but the staff are not. So it is usually easier for you to adapt to their systems rather than the other way round.

○ If the pharmacy employs well trained dispensing technicians, it may be more efficient for them to produce labels, simply because they are used to the computer system. Indeed, depending on the number of staff and the workload in a particular pharmacy, you may prefer to spend little time in the dispensary and devote most of your day to advising and counselling patients and customers. If you do need to familiarise yourself with a new system, aim to do this during quieter periods of the day.

○ If you cannot find something, ask rather than waste time looking for it yourself.

○ Check with staff exactly when they would like help, e.g. putting away orders.

○ If you have to leave the pharmacy area even for a short time, tell a member of staff so that they do not have to chase round looking for you when a prescription comes in or you need to speak to a customer.

○ If you need to make any personal telephone calls, mention that you are doing so and offer to pay. Alternatively, use your own mobile phone or a telephone charge card with which call charges are billed to you personally.

WHERE TO GET HELP

Few days in a pharmacy run completely smoothly, but you will be able to sort out most minor difficulties yourself or by asking a member of the staff. However, it is often useful to know where you can obtain further help, and this will obviously depend on the nature of the problem.

Many of your queries about prescriptions such as those relating to the requirements of the Drug Tariff (e.g. prescription endorsement, allowable and non-allowable items on the NHS); Controlled Drug regulations; how and where to obtain unusual products can be answered by the NPA's information department.

The Royal Pharmaceutical Society's law department will clarify legal issues. Their information department will do searches and provide copies of journal articles, for which they make a charge. You can also borrow books from the library – they will send them by post.

Remember that when you work as a locum, you are not just looking after the professional side of things, but you are also looking after a shop and a property with all the problems that can occur as a result of this – shoplifting, burglary, broken windows, floods, breakdown of equipment, and so on. If you are doing a locum for a multiple and you experience a problem like this, the usual procedure will be to ring the company's head office. Most companies leave emergency telephone numbers in the pharmacy, so if a difficulty occurs in the evening or at the weekend, you have someone to contact.

If you are working for an independent, make sure that you have an emergency contact. If the proprietor has gone away on holiday, this may not be possible. Try to make sure that you have emergency contact numbers for a local electrician, plumber and glazier and for the police, fire service, burglar alarm and pharmacy computer.

LOCKING UP

Always stay in the evening until the shop is secure, whether or not you are a key holder. If it is dark, ask the staff how they intend to get home. If necessary, offer a lift. They will appreciate you asked even if their arrangements are satisfactory. If you are going on to a different pharmacy the next day, make sure that you have left full explanatory notes of any unusual occurrences, including special orders, customer complaints, shoplifting etc., and that you have left a contact number for the next day or two.

5

Dispensing

This chapter provides some brief guidance on dispensing practice and procedure in community pharmacy. Despite current and expected future changes in pharmacy practice, dispensing remains the focus of much of your work as a locum.

This chapter aims to highlight important points in dispensing practice, especially those which if you have not practised for a while, are easy to overlook. It is by no means comprehensive and if you feel you need further guidance, particularly on legal and ethical issues, please refer to *Medicines Ethics and Practice* (see also Appendix 1).

A systematic approach in dealing with prescriptions (see Table 5.1) is vital. This is particularly important when you are working in unfamiliar surroundings.

As part of this structured approach, several points are worth highlighting, particularly if you are new to community pharmacy or have had a long break from it.

O   Check the patient's name and address and if the pharmacy employs a docket system, use it.

O   Before dispensing a prescription, sort out whether the patient pays or is exempt and make sure that the back of the prescription is properly filled in.

O   About 80 per cent of patients are exempt from charges. These include patients who are: under the age of 16; 16–19 years but in full-time education; over the age of 60; in receipt of Income

Table 5.1 Dealing with prescriptions

---

1 Receive the prescription from the patient (or the patient's representative), and make sure the relevant sections on the back of the prescription are completed.

2 Think about the patient for whom you are dispensing the prescription and consider the appropriateness of the medicine, the dose and the instructions and assessing the possibility of drug interactions and adverse drug reactions.

3 Check that the medicines are in stock.

4 Prepare a label.

5 Dispense the medicines.

6 Issue the prescription to the patient (or the patient's representative) with appropriate information and advice about the medicines.

7 Endorse the prescription – the computer may do this for you, but check that it has done so correctly.

8 Make any necessary records.

9 File the prescription.

Support, Family Credit or Disability Allowance; holders of various exemption (including pre-payment) certificates.

○ If a patient wishes to claim back a prescription charge, use the special form (FP57), which should be kept in the pharmacy.

○ When dealing with NHS prescriptions, check for: items which attract multiple charges (e.g. some hormone replacement therapy products); items which look as if they might attract multiple charges (e.g. several flavours of one product), but are in fact a single charge and other unusual charges (e.g. hosiery); and items which are not allowed on the NHS. Get to know the Drug Tariff and use the *NPA Guide to the Drug Tariff* to help you.

○ Watch out for unusual items or unusual quantities and check whether you have sufficient stock.

○ Check for items which are not allowed (the 'Black List') on NHS prescriptions. The dispensary computer will usually tell you this when you enter a blacklisted item. In addition, details of all products included in the Black List can be found in the Drug Tariff or the *BNF*.

○ Check the date on the prescription. Prescriptions are valid for six months unless they are for Controlled Drugs (Schedule 2 and 3), in which case they are valid for 13 weeks.

○ Check the patient's age if under 12 years; this is essential for checking the dose.

○ Check the patient's medication record for possible incompatibilities with the new prescription.

○ For Controlled Drugs, every legally required detail (see Table 5.2) must be hand written by the prescriber.

○ If the item is one that needs re-constituting, diluting or preparing extemporaneously, check that the quantity ordered will not last longer than the 'shelf life'.

○ Preparing the label before dispensing the medicine helps you to concentrate on the prescribed instructions; this may highlight some problem that you have not spotted so far (e.g. an unusual dose or quantity).

○ Destroy all surplus or unwanted labels from the printer roll immediately; this prevents the inadvertent use of incorrect labels.

○ Remember to put leaflets, spoons and measures as appropriate with the finished medicine.

Table 5.2 Summary of Controlled Drug regulations*

Schedule	2 CD	3 CDNoReg	4 CD Anab; CD Benz	5 CDInv
Handwriting requirements[1]	Yes	Yes, except temazepam & phenobarbitone[2]	No	No
Validity of prescription	13 weeks	13 weeks	6 months	6 months
Address of prescriber in UK?[3]	Yes	Yes	No	No
Safe custody	Yes (except quinalbarbitone)	No (except buprenorphine diethylpropion, temazepam)	No	No
Emergency supplies allowed?	No	No (except phenobarbitone for epilepsy)	Yes	Yes
Dispensing by instalments (NHS prescriptions)	Yes	No	No	No
Repeats allowed?[4]	No	No	Yes	Yes
Entry in CD register?	Yes	No	No	No
'CD' endorsement (NHS prescriptions)	Yes	Yes	No	No
Mark date of supply on prescription (NHS)	Yes	Yes	No	No
Stock destruction to be witnessed	Yes	No	No	No
Requisitions necessary	Yes	Yes	No	No
Invoices to be retained for 2 years?	No	Yes	No, except for anabolic steroids	Yes
Licences required for import and export?	Yes	Yes	No, except for anabolic steroids	No

Notes
1 The following must be specified in the prescriber's own handwriting: patient's name and address (or for a veterinary prescription, the person to whom the CD is to be delivered); dose, form and strength; total quantity in words and figures.
2 Prescriptions for phenobarbitone do not have to be written in the doctor's own handwriting. However, the dose, form and strength must be present and the total quantity written in words and figures. The prescription must be signed and dated by the prescriber. Temazepam is exempt from all the prescription and handwriting CD regulations.
3 The UK does not include the Channel Islands or the Isle of Man.
4 If a Controlled Drug is Schedule 4 or 5 and prescribed on a repeatable basis, the first supply must be made within six months of the prescription being issued.

NB: Schedule 2 CDs include the opiates and quinalbarbitone, Schedule 3 contains most of the barbiturates and temazepam, Schedule 4 the anabolic steroids and benzodiazepines and Schedule 5 contains many of the drugs listed in Schedule 2, but in restricted strengths, certain pharmaceutical forms and often in combination with other substances (see *Medicines Ethics and Practice* for precise details of CD schedules).
*Adapted from NPA information leaflet *Controlled Drugs and Community Pharmacy*

O   Double check the patient's name and address when giving out dispensed medicines, even if the pharmacy uses a docket system.

O   If you are unsure about anything on the prescription, contact the prescriber.

O   It may be worth advising the pharmacy staff and the patients that you may be a little slower than the regular pharmacist, at least until you find your feet.

FORGED PRESCRIPTIONS

Be on your guard for forged prescriptions. Check whether any notification of stolen prescription forms has been received at the pharmacy. Doctors who have had forms stolen often write subsequent prescriptions in red or green ink for a while. If the prescription turns out to be a forgery, telephone the police. In addition, contact the local health authority or local pharmaceutical committee (LPC) so that they can alert other pharmacies. They will also give you details of any local policy.

TYPES OF NHS PRESCRIPTIONS

Be aware that there are several types of NHS prescriptions. The most commonly used is the white FP10, but others include:

O   FP14 (yellow) dental prescriptions. Remember that dentists can only prescribe from a limited range of items. These items are listed in the *BNF* and the Drug Tariff.

○ FP10(HP) (orange or dark red) hospital prescriptions.

○ FP10 (MDA) (blue) double-sided prescriptions for addicts (used by GPs).

○ FP10 (HP)(Ad) (pink) double-sided prescriptions for addicts used by licensed medical practitioners working at addiction clinics or from hospital outpatient departments (see below for details about dispensing for drug misusers).

○ FP296 and FMED296 (buff or sand coloured) forces prescriptions.

○ FP10 (DTS) drug testing scheme forms. These are used by Royal Pharmaceutical Society inspectors. If you have a visit from an inspector he or she will probably want to take a sample of a dispensed prescription for testing. The FP10(DTS) allows you to dispense a new supply for the patient. One copy of this form should be kept with the part of the sample left by the inspector in the pharmacy.

PRIVATE PRESCRIPTIONS

Private prescriptions sometimes cause a bit of difficulty, simply because pharmacists tend to deal with them less frequently than with NHS prescriptions. Full details can be found in *Medicines, Ethics and Practice*, but the main points to watch out for when dispensing private prescriptions are as follows:

○ Prescriptions for prescription-only medicines (POMs) are valid six months after the date of issue.

○ If the prescription is repeatable, it must be dispensed for the first time within six months of the date on the prescription.

○ Prescriptions must be retained for two years.

○ There is no limit to the number of repeats that the prescriber can put on the prescription, but if it just says 'repeat', then the prescription can only be repeated once, i.e. first dispensing and one repeat only.

○ Controlled Drugs may NOT be repeated (see Table 5.2), but can, at the direction of the prescriber, be dispensed in instalments on specified dates.

○ When the final repeat has been dispensed, the pharmacy dispensing the final supply must keep the prescription for two years.

○ If there are other items on a repeat prescription that can be repeated but ONE of the items has been supplied in full, the pharmacist who has dispensed the complete item MUST keep the prescription.

○ An appropriate entry must be made in the Private Prescription Book. A record is only legally required for a POM medicine, but it is good practice to keep records of all private prescriptions.

○ The prescription must be stamped and dated with the pharmacy stamp. A reference number corresponding to the record in the prescription book must be written on the prescription. If it is a repeat prescription, you need to stamp the prescription each time you dispense it and write down the number of times the prescription has been dispensed.

Each pharmacy generally has a policy for charging for private prescriptions. Find out what this is, if possible. Many pharmacies have a set formula, such as cost of the item plus 50 per cent and sometimes a fee on top of this. Some pharmacists have a minimum charge, some charge an extra fee for Controlled Drugs and some operate a different pricing policy for high-cost items than for low-cost items. Remember that private prescriptions do NOT attract Value Added Tax (VAT).

CONTROLLED DRUGS

Controlled Drugs often cause you problems as a locum, particularly if you are unfamiliar with the doctors' signatures and the patients. Added to which, problems often occur late in the evening or on Saturday afternoon when you cannot get hold of the prescriber. If you are unsatisfied as to whether a prescription is genuine, start by looking through the prescriptions which have already been dispensed and filed away. You may be fortunate enough to find another prescription written by the same doctor, so enabling you to check the doctor's signature. Look in the Controlled Drugs register and see if the patient has had the Controlled Drug before and how frequently. Ask a member of staff if he or she knows the patient and doctor concerned.

If you are still unsatisfied as to whether the prescription is genuine, you may wish to contact the prescriber. If you do not know the doctor, check their telephone number with Directory Enquiries or the Health Authority/Health Board list and make sure the doctor is licensed to prescribe Controlled Drugs. Other sources of information about the medical register include the Royal Pharmaceutical Society, the National Pharmaceutical Association and the General Medical Council (see Appendix 2).

If a CD prescription is incorrectly written but you are 100 per cent satisfied that the prescription is genuine and that the patient is in immediate need of it, you will have to exercise your professional judgement as to whether or not to supply it. If you are not going to be at the pharmacy the next day, always leave full explanatory notes, but if you decide to dispense the item, the final responsibility rests with you.

A summary of the regulations for the supply of Controlled Drugs is shown in Table 5.2. For further details, see the NPA information leaflet *Controlled Drugs and Community Pharmacy*.

DISPENSING FOR DRUG MISUSERS

Full details of the regulations for dispensing prescriptions for drug misusers can be found in the NPA leaflet *Controlled Drugs and Community Pharmacy*. Remember in particular that there are two types of prescriptions for addicts (pink and blue – see above) and that the prescription requirements are the same as those shown in Table 5.2. Important points to highlight include the following:

○ The most commonly prescribed drug for addicts is methadone, and prescriptions are usually written for instalment dispensing.

○ The drugs are usually ordered to be dispensed daily and the doctor must indicate the amount to be dispensed on each instalment as well as the interval between instalments.

○ Double amounts are usually prescribed to take account of Sundays and public holidays.

○ Only doctors licensed by the Home Office can prescribe cocaine, diamorphine and dipipanone for the treatment of addicts.

○ You must dispense the drug on the date on which it is due.

○   Instalments not dispensed on the right day cannot be collected on a later day.

○   Drugs must always be collected by the addict personally, unless another arrangement has been made with the pharmacy.

○   After dispensing, you must endorse the prescription in the space provided with the date, the amount supplied and your initials and you must also make an entry in the CD register.

Some pharmacists are now supervising the self-administration of methadone because patients cannot necessarily be relied upon to take it, and a great deal of methadone therefore ends up on the black market. If you work as a locum in a pharmacy which supervises method administration, there are several points to consider:

○   Measuring out the methadone, pouring it into a cup and giving the cup to the patients contravenes the Medicines Act regarding the labelling of dispensed medicines. This is because dispensing and administration of medicines are two separate processes. You must therefore dispense the medicine into a labelled bottle in the usual manner. The patient can then take the dose from the labelled bottle or you can pour it from that bottle into a cup.

○   Check that patients have actually taken the methadone (e.g. talk to them afterwards or get them to swallow a glassful of water in front of you).

It is also worth obtaining a copy of *Pharmaceutical Aspects of Methadone Prescribing* from the Scottish Centre for Pharmacy Postgraduate Education (SCPPE; telephone: 0141 552 4400, extension 4273/4). This distance learning pack is free if you work in Scotland, but costs £12 if you work elsewhere. However, you can borrow it free of charge if you live anywhere in the UK.

PARALLEL IMPORTS

Parallel imports are branded products that are imported or re-imported from Europe. The reason that parallel imports exist is that some drugs are sold cheaper in Europe than the UK. However, the price received by the pharmacist for dispensing these products is based on the going rate in the UK. So, there is a financial incentive for supplying them.

If you work in a pharmacy where parallel imports are used, always check that:

○ The products have a Product Licence (PL) or a Parallel Importing Product Licence (PI) number clearly stated on the pack. Pharmacists who buy or supply unlicensed products are open to disciplinary action for unprofessional conduct.

○ The generic name on the foreign product is the same as that used in the UK.

○ All the necessary information and labelling on the product is in English. This information can be in other languages as well.

Problems occur when the licensed imported product has a different brand name to the British product. For example, Voltaren tablets (a parallel import) may be supplied against prescriptions for diclofenac, but not against prescriptions for Voltarol. When a brand name is prescribed, you must always supply that brand. This may mean that you have to order a small amount to cover a supply.

EMERGENCY SUPPLIES

Patients may sometimes ask if they can have a supply of a prescription-only medicine without having a prescription. They may have run out of their medication, forgotten to bring their medication out with them or they may have developed a problem for which they have been prescribed the medication in the past. Guidelines for making emergency supplies can be found in *Medicines, Ethics and Practice*. These guidelines focus on one main consideration; that is, what would be the medical consequences of not supplying? You must use your professional judgement, and asking the patient the following questions will help you to make a decision:

○ Has the patient had a prescription for this problem within the last six months?

○ Is it impossible for the patient to obtain a prescription immediately?

○ Will the condition get significantly worse if not treated today?

Remember that if you decide to make an emergency supply, this must be done in accordance with the law (see *Medicines, Ethics and Practice*), and various records are required.

LENDING TABLETS

Locums are often faced with patients who ask if they can borrow medicines. A patient may tell you that 'the normal pharmacist always gives me a few tablets'. Again, it is down to your professional judgement. Be aware of the legal requirements for making emergency supplies to patients. If you decide to charge for the medication, the patient may not be too pleased. One way round the charging issue is to charge the patient anyway and ask the patient to keep the receipt and to take it up with the proprietor when he or she returns from holiday.

6

Computers

When you do a locum in a pharmacy for the first time, it may be the thought of an unfamiliar computer system that worries you most. There are several pharmacy computer systems, but probably about half a dozen fairly common ones. Every system is slightly different, but there are some basic features common to all of them. These include the facility to:

○ Generate and print labels.

○ Generate patient medication records.

○ Order and manage stock (see Chapter 7).

Several pharmacies also use their computers for leaflet production and Electronic Point of Sale (EPoS) recording of sales information. The introduction of computer technology represents a huge investment for proprietors, and for it to produce meaningful information, it must be used systematically and according to strict discipline. For example, quantities must be entered correctly. Patient names should always be entered in the same way. If you enter S Holt on one occasion and Susie Holt on another, you will have two records for the same patient. Make sure, therefore, that you learn as soon as possible how to delete any information which you have entered incorrectly.

PRODUCING LABELS

Pharmacy computer systems may produce several types of labels, including those for dispensed and over-the-counter medicines, address labels for bags and owing slips.

To produce a label for a dispensed medicine, the procedure will probably be close to the following:

○ You usually start with the patient's name. This normally involves typing three or four letters of the surname or sometimes the full surname and perhaps an initial. If the patient is already recorded on the computer, s/he may give you a patient registration card which may include a number. Sometimes you can type in this number to find the patient on the patient medication record. (Indeed if the patient is on the PMR and you are supplying repeats of previous items, it is just a matter of identifying those items on the computer, checking that the details are correct and generating a repeat label.)

○ The drug details come next. Sometimes you type the drug name in first, sometimes the quantity on the prescription. For drugs, you generally type in the first three or four letters. A menu of drugs beginning with those letters will appear on the screen and you select the drug (with its strength, if appropriate) written on the prescription.

○ For the quantity, it is normally a matter of typing in the appropriate number. Most computer systems have a facility for typing in numbers of packs. So, for example, if you want to dispense a tube of cream, you normally type in 1 and not 30 g. Similarly with contraceptives; for three months' supply, you might just need to type in 3, or if it is a triple pack, you might just type in 1. If you type in two packs, you will get two labels etc. But some systems do use other methods for generating more than one label. If you dispense two packs with different quantities in them, the correct quantities must be put on each label.

○ Generating the directions for using the medicine usually involves the use of codes. Once you have used a few systems, you can usually guess what the codes will be. Thus, one three times a day is normally 1T or some variation on that. If you are completely unfamiliar with a system, find the computer instruction book which will list all the appropriate codes. Some pharmacies keep a list of these codes next to the computer itself.

○ Cautionary labels and warnings will normally appear automatically.

○ The system will normally allow you to amend labels and re-print them without disturbing the patient's record. Try and learn how to do this as soon as possible.

○ There will probably be a facility to record any item(s) or part items you owe to a patient. Not only will a record remain on the computer data base, but the computer will also generate an extra label(s) for you to give to the patient as part of an owings slip.

○ Most systems give you the opportunity to free type anything extra or unusual.

PATIENT MEDICATION RECORDS

Most pharmacies now keep patient medication records (PMRs) on their computers. Effectively a data base, the PMR can be a complete record of both prescription and OTC medicines supplied to each patient. In practice, however, patients go to more than one pharmacy and there is never a guarantee that the record kept in one pharmacy is accurate and complete.

If, while working as a locum you need to generate a new PMR, it is usually a matter of starting with the patient's name. Indeed, the system will tell you whether that particular patient is on record or not, and if not, the option to create a record will normally appear on the computer screen. Remember that confidentiality is an important issue when creating PMRs. Information about patients held in computer systems is subject to the Data Protection Act and in line with this Act, information entered in a PMR should be volunteered by, or obtained from, the patient concerned. Creating a PMR involves keying in the following types of data:

○ The patient's details, e.g. name, address (or name of residential home), telephone number, NHS number, sex, date of birth, exemption from prescription charges.

○ General practitioner details, e.g. name, practice name, telephone number.

○ Dispensed medicines, including name, strength, form, quantity, dose and date of dispensing.

○ Chronic illnesses/conditions (e.g. asthma, diabetes), allergies, drug sensitivities (e.g. aspirin, penicillin).

○ The brand of medicine preferred or colour or manufacturer of generic.

○ The acceptability or otherwise of child-resistant closures to the patient.

○ Medication requiring particular vigilance (e.g. warfarin).

○ Whether the patient is pregnant or breast-feeding

One major advantage of PMRs is the ability to generate repeat labels. You can, of course, alter any of the information in a PMR to produce the label you need. The repeat label facility is particularly useful for servicing residential and nursing homes and dispensing medicines in monitored dosage systems and for repeat prescription services, including collection and delivery services.

SWITCHING OFF THE COMPUTER

Many computer programs hold information in Random Access Memory (RAM), information which will be lost when the computer is switched off. Check before switching off whether any data held in memory needs to be saved either on to a disc or a tape. Also check if the data should be copied in any case; this provides a secure back-up, should a fault develop in the computer.

7

Ordering stock

Stock control and management are an important part of running a pharmacy, even if you are only there for a day. Indeed, finding out about the pharmacy's ordering systems is something you should try and do as early on your first day as possible. At the very least, make sure you find out about:

○ Delivery times – you will need to let patients know when out of stock or owing items will be available for collection.

○ How much in advance orders need to be placed. When are the deadlines?

○ The method of ordering. For example, is it automated? Is the pharmacy computer linked directly by modem to one or more wholesalers? Do you have to phone orders through to the wholesaler? Or does the wholesaler phone you?

THE ORDERING PROCESS

Many pharmacies these days order stock via their computers. The computer is likely to allow you to order stock in three ways:

○ Manually during labelling.

○ Manually outside of the labelling process.

○ Automatically while dispensing.

Ordering manually on the computer normally involves typing the first three or four letters of the drug name OR some sort of a code such as the Pharmaceutical Interface Product (PIP) code, which is seven numbers and unique to each product, OR the wholesaler's order number. There will also be a facility for amending orders, say, if you've ordered too much of an item or too little or the wrong item.

The computer may be set to order automatically. Check if this is the case. When you enter the amount of a drug to produce a medicine label, the computer calculates from pre-set figures whether or not more stock is required. However, if you make a mistake when typing in drug quantities, you will need to alter stock figures. If you are unsure how to do this, keep the incorrect labels to one side and if you leave the pharmacy without being able to adjust the stock figures, leave a note for the owner or manager of the quantities to be adjusted.

If the pharmacy has more than one supplier, drugs listed on the computer may be automatically linked to one supplier or another. With some systems you may have to do this for yourself, i.e. decide which supplier you wish to order from. Check, in particular, what happens to the orders for over-the-counter medicines and generics and how appliances and dressings are ordered.

ORDER TRANSMISSION

Orders can generally be transmitted in one of two ways:

○ Via a modem from the pharmacy computer to the wholesaler's computer terminal.

○ By telephone.

Check whether orders sent off to wholesalers via the computer are automatically cancelled. If not, they will need to be cancelled or the order will be sent twice and charged twice.

RECEIVING ORDERS

When orders arrive, there are several checks which you should make, most of which are common sense. The first and most important check is that the parcel, box, or plastic tray is for the pharmacy you are working in. Do this before the driver leaves the pharmacy. If you are busy, it is all too easy to sign for goods only to find out later that they are for another pharmacy.

If Controlled Drugs are included in the delivery, you must make a full check of these and sign for them. CDs should be locked away without delay and the appropriate entries made in the CD register.

When checking off orders make sure that:

○ The item is correct (against the invoice and/or delivery note).

○ The pack size is correct.

○ The number of packs or bottles is correct.

○ The pack is undamaged.

○ The expiry date is acceptable.

○ The item is not subject to special storage requirements. Wholesalers often put items for the refrigerator in separate bags. Identify these and put them away immediately (see also Table 7.1).

Table 7.1 Items required to be stored in the refrigerator

Achromycin powder	Insulin preparations	Pancrex V preparations
Achromycin ointment	Ketovite preparations	Pro-Actidil tablets
Alkeran tablets	Ledercort cream	Restandol capsules (once
Aureocort cream	Leukeran tablets	opened store at room
Aureomycin cream/	Medihaler – ergotamine	temperature, shelf life
ointment/ophthalmic	Miacalcic Minims	three months)
ointment	Mydrilate eye drops	Sno-Phenicol
Chloramphenicol eye drops	Myerlan 0.5 mg tablets	Sno-Pilo
Daktacort cream	Neosporin eye drops	Timodine cream
Eppy eye drops	Nystatin powder	Varidase
Heminevrin syrup	Otosporin ear drops	Vaccines

The dispensary refrigerator is capable of storing products between 2 and 8°C. Check the temperature regularly, particularly if you are working in one pharmacy for a few days, and if you ever find it outside of the correct temperature range, get the refrigerator checked immediately. Remember also to check with product manufacturers to see if any of the products in the refrigerator could have deteriorated

---

In addition, find out whether:

O   Records of deliveries are kept on the computer or elsewhere. Some pharmacies check the invoices and file them away. Others, however, book deliveries into the computer and possibly also into a delivery book. Check whether this is the case and if so, find out how to complete these records. You may also need to sign or initial the delivery note/invoice to say that the goods have arrived. Finally, file the invoice away.

O   There are special procedures for returning stock. If you want to send any stock back (e.g. it has been ordered in error, the wholesaler has sent too much, stock is damaged, product or batch recall by the manufacturer), deal with this immediately. Most wholesalers give their customers a special book for recording details of returned stock. A credit note or an invoice adjustment will appear later.

8

Additional pharmacy services

Many community pharmacists offer several additional services, and as a locum, the ones you are most likely to be involved in include pregnancy testing, needle exchange schemes, collection and delivery of prescriptions and monitored dosage systems. This chapter highlights the main points which are likely to affect your work as a locum in these areas.

You should also make sure that you know how to measure and fit surgical hosiery and trusses. (The NPA runs a course on truss fitting, which you can access if you work in an NPA member's pharmacy.) You may also need to know about supplying and delivering oxygen. There is no substitute for visiting a patient with an experienced pharmacist or technician to demonstrate the correct procedures. In addition, *Medicines Ethics and Practice* gives guidelines on oxygen.

PREGNANCY TESTING IN THE PHARMACY

Many community pharmacies offer a pregnancy testing service (in addition to selling self-testing kits). The test procedure itself is normally very easy to follow, but the following additional points should be borne in mind:

O   The woman (who wants to know whether or not she is pregnant) should herself request the test.

○ You should fill in the appropriate form with, for example, the woman's name, address and the name of her doctor before you do the test.

○ Cover any cuts and grazes on your hands with a waterproof dressing.

○ Carry out the test on a shelf next to the wash basin in the toilet (if possible).

○ Wash your hands after doing the test.

○ Record the results on the form.

○ Keep a copy of the result.

○ Give the results to the patient (not to anyone else).

○ Tip the urine sample down the toilet.

NEEDLE AND SYRINGE EXCHANGE SCHEMES

You may find yourself working in a pharmacy which provides a service to drug misusers in which needles and syringes are supplied on an exchange basis. There should also be a local counselling service available for drug misusers to obtain advice on safe needle use and safe sex.

The Royal Pharmaceutical Society has produced guidelines for pharmacists involved in needle exchange. These guidelines are reproduced in full in *Medicines Ethics and Practice*. Those that are relevant to the return of needles and syringes are as follows:

○ Always dispose of dirty needles and syringes through a recognised sharps disposal scheme.

○ You should NOT touch used syringes and needles. The user should bring them to the pharmacy in an outer container and then put them straight into the sharps disposal box.

○ The sharps box should be stored in a secure place (well away from customers) and made available for the user to deposit syringes and needles.

If you work in pharmacies where you deal frequently with drug misusers, it may be worthwhile considering having a hepatitis vaccination.

COLLECTION AND DELIVERY SERVICES

Some patients may experience difficulty in obtaining prescriptions, particularly if they live in geographically isolated areas, and are disabled, ill or elderly. In order to meet the needs of these people, pharmacies often operate collection and delivery schemes – collection of repeat prescriptions, usually from the patients' surgeries, and delivery of the dispensed items, usually and preferably to the patients' homes. A patient's home may, of course, be a nursing or residential home. As a locum, you may be involved in collection and delivery of prescriptions. Full guidance for collection and delivery services can be found in *Medicines, Ethics and Practice*, but the following points should be borne in mind:

○ The request for such a service must come from the patient or carer. The pharmacist must not initiate the service for an individual patient. Patients must give their consent to a prescription being directed to a particular pharmacy.

○ The pharmacy must operate a patient medication record (PMR) system, which must be registered with the Data Protection Register.

○ The prescriber must indicate the length of time for which the repeats can be continued. On dispensing the final repeat, the pharmacist must remind patients in writing that they need to visit their doctor.

○ Pharmacists may not ask for a repeat prescription for a patient even if that patient normally has the service from that pharmacy. The request must come from the patient.

○ Patients must tell the pharmacist which from their list of medications they require. Check the PMR and make sure that the patient is ordering repeats appropriately. For example, a month's supply of a salbutamol inhaler may be lasting less than two weeks or a month's supply of diuretics may be lasting for three weeks.

○ Always give the medicines to the patient or carer.

○ Never leave medicines with a neighbour unless the patient has told you to do this.

MONITORED DOSAGE SYSTEMS

You may work in pharmacies which provide monitored dosage systems, and if you have not worked in community pharmacy before or have been away from it for several years, MDS will probably be quite new to you. Pharmacies which are busy with MDS often have a separate area for this activity and a trained technician to fill the trays. Beyond supervising the dispensing and checking the drug records you will not have to worry. However, if the pharmacy has just a few patients on MDS, you may have to fill the trays yourself. Find out if this is the case and try to familiarise yourself with the system before you have to do it on your own.

Monitored dosage systems are designed to make giving medication, easy, safe and hygienic and to take up less time than giving medicines from ordinary containers. They are used principally in nursing and residential homes. Medicines are dispensed into plastic trays with separate slots for different times of day, different days of the week and depending on the system, different weeks of the month. Patients (or their carers) can check that the medicine has been taken at the right time and in the right amount and that nothing has been missed.

There are basically two types of systems on the market:

○ Rigid cassettes (e.g. Nomad).

○ Foil and blister systems (e.g. Manrex).

Cassettes

All the medicines for one dosage time (e.g. morning or night) are placed in one compartment of the tray. Thus, if the patient takes one bendrofluazide 2.5 mg tablet and one atenolol 50 mg tablet, both in the morning, each tablet will be put in one compartment. The Nomad system holds a week's supply of each medicine.

Foil and blister systems

In this system, there are completely separate trays for doses taken at different times of day. So, for example you might have a tray for morning doses, one for lunch-time doses, one for teatime or evening doses, one for bedtime doses and one for PRN (when required) doses. In the Manrex system, the trays are colour coded to correspond to the timing of the doses. So, all morning doses might go in a pink tray, lunch-time doses in a yellow tray, teatime doses in an orange tray, bedtime doses in a blue tray and PRN doses in a white tray etc.

Each tray holds 28 days' worth of medication. Each dose is placed in one of the 28 bubbles in the blister packaging, sealed with foil and then the pack placed in a plastic tray of the appropriate colour.

Medicine administration record (MAR) charts

Both types of MDS system employ medicine administration record (MAR) charts. MAR charts are usually generated on the pharmacy computer (from the patient medication record), using three-part paper as follows:

O   The top copy serves as the medication record in the home.

O   The second copy is used for medication review.

O   The third copy is used for re-ordering the medication.

DISPENSING MDS

As for other areas of pharmacy practice, it is important to follow certain procedures (for further details, see *Medicines, Ethics and Practice*). Particular points you should remember include:

○ Dispensing MDS must be supervised by a pharmacist.

○ Any changes to the medication regimens and MAR charts must be supervised by the pharmacist.

○ Ideally, the pharmacy should have a separate area (with enough space for all the equipment) for assembling MDS; the area should be clean, tidy and hygienic.

○ Medicines should NOT be left in sealed monitored dosage systems for longer than eight weeks.

○ Tablets and capsules which are hard to tell apart should NOT be put into one compartment of the MDS.

○ After filling, the MDS should be protected from light and stored in a cool, dry place.

○ Homes should return any unwanted medicines to the pharmacy.

In addition, bear in mind that certain types of medication should NOT be dispensed in MDS. These are:

○ Effervescent and dispersible tablets.

○ Buccal and sublingual tablets.

○ Cytotoxics.

○ Liquids.

○ Suppositories, pessaries, eye/ear drops etc.

○ Tablets and capsules which must be dispensed in their original container.

○ With some MDS (e.g. Nomad), PRN dosages are NOT put into MDS trays.

9

Income tax matters

As soon as you start to work as a locum, you should inform your local inspector of taxes. Find the Inland Revenue in the local phone directory and ask them to send you the following booklets:

○ "Self Assessment – A general guide".

○ "Starting your own business?" (CWL1).

As well as giving useful tax and National Insurance contributions information, CWL1 contains two forms, first, CWF1 (coloured green) which is required for notifying the Inland Revenue and the Contributions Agency of your self-employed status and second, the form CA5601 (peach coloured), which you should fill in if you wish to pay your National Insurance contributions by direct debit.

In addition, ask for a Schedule D reference number. The NPA advises its members to ask locums for this number as evidence of tax status. Otherwise members may find themselves in dispute with the Inland Revenue.

If you have left your previous employment, you should send to your local Inspector of Taxes parts 2 and 3 of your P45 form provided by your last employer, but keep part 1A for your own records. If you do locums in addition to either full or part-time regular employment, your employer will keep your P45. However, you must declare your locum earnings on your tax return.

Your main task as far as income tax is concerned is completing a tax return, and to do this you need to keep good records.

RECORDS

The first thing to do is to draw up an account book or buy a ready made one from a stationery shop. Alternatively, you may decide to keep your accounts on a computer, using one of the personal financial packages now available. Keep all your entries simple and logical. Make a clear record of all transactions, both incomings and outgoings. Keep a note of business and personal mileage, and if you do not have a separate business telephone line, make a note of all business calls.

Retain all your receipts and copies of invoices. This is because all entries on your tax return must be supported by appropriate documentation. Moreover, you must keep all your records for five years after the deadline for sending in your tax return. And if you receive other income from for example, renting a property, you must keep all documentation relevant to that for five years too. If the Revenue wants to audit your accounts, you must keep your records until the audit is complete, even if this is longer than the normal period. The Revenue will not normally ask to see supporting documents, but if they do, and you have not kept them, there are some heavy penalties.

TAX RETURNS

The tax year runs from April 6 of one year until April 5 in the following year and you will need to fill in a tax return at the end of each tax year. The tax return must be submitted by:

○ January 31 following the end of the tax year; or

○ Three months after the date of issue of the tax return if this is later.

When you receive your tax return form, you will notice that it is divided into two main parts both of which you need to complete. In the first section, you identify exactly what you have earned and from which sources as well as capital gains, reliefs, deductions and allowances for the tax year. In the second section you calculate your tax bill. This is known as self-assessment. Until April 1996, the Inland Revenue used to calculate your income tax from your tax return and then send you a tax bill. However, calculation of your tax bill is now your responsibility, unless you specify otherwise (see below).

There are three methods of calculating your tax liability. You can:

○ Do it yourself.

○ Ask your accountant to do it for you.

○ Ask the Inspector of Taxes to do it, but your tax return must be submitted by September 30 in the same year as the end of the relevant tax year. However, if the Revenue sends you your tax return after August 1, you can send it to them for calculation of your tax bill, but you must do this within two months of the date of issue.

If you wish to calculate your own tax, you must send in a tax return by January 31 in the year following the tax year.

Returns not sent in by that date will incur a penalty of £100, and returns still outstanding six months later will incur a further penalty of £100. There are more penalties for incorrect or fraudulent returns.

If you do not include a self assessment with a tax return submitted after September 30, the Revenue has the power to issue the assessment on your behalf. You would then have to pay the tax based on that assessment. But the Revenue does not guarantee to do the calculations before you are due to pay the tax if you send the return after September 30. So you could have to pay interest and, possibly, surcharges.

INCOME TAX RATES

Income tax rates for 1996/7 are shown in Table 9.1.

TAX DEDUCTIBLE EXPENSES

Tax deductible expenses include:

O   Your RPSGB annual fees, plus any other professional subscriptions.

O   Business telephone bills (including mobile telephone).

O   Capital allowances for cost of desk, answering machine, fax machine, computer and other office equipment.

O   Stationery and postage.

O   Overalls.

O   Travel expenses, including car purchase and running costs.

Table 9.1 Income tax rates and allowances (1998/9)

Lower	20%	Up to £4300
Basic	23%	£4300–27 100
Upper	40%	Above £27 100
Allowances		
Personal allowance		£4195
Married couple's allowance		£1900
Age allowance (65–74)		
Personal allowance		£5410
Married couple's allowance		£3305
Age allowances (75 and over)		
Personal allowance		£5600
Married couple's allowance		£3345
Income limit for age allowance		£16 200

○ Accountant's fees.

○ Textbooks and relevant journals.

○ Meeting and conference fees.

○ Depreciation and repair costs (for relevant items).

○ Professional indemnity insurance fees.

○ A proportion of your household expenses such as heat and light to cover your office space.

PAYING YOUR TAX

You have to make three payments to the Inland Revenue for each tax year. Considering the tax year 1998/9 as an illustration, you would need to make:

○ Two payments on account – one on January 31 1999 and the other on July 31 1999.

○ One payment of remaining tax on 31 January 2000.

The two payments on account are usually equal amounts of money and are calculated as your total tax liability for the previous tax year (in the above example, this would be the tax year 1997/8), less any income tax deducted at source for that year. You will not have to make any payments on account if the amounts due are less than minimum limits set by the Revenue. For example, if you have a full-time job and pay most of your tax by PAYE, your additional tax liability for a few days' locums may fall below the threshold, and you will not have to pay anything on account.

You may think that you should pay less than the required payment on account. For example, if your tax liability for 1997/8 was £4000, your payments on account for 1998/9 will be: £2000 on 31 January 1999 and £2000 on 31 July 1999. However, if you consider you tax liability for 1998/9 to be £3000, you can write to the Inland Revenue and claim to reduce your two payments on account to £1500 each.

Any further tax due (after the two payments on account) must be paid by January 31 in the following year. If you do not pay your tax on time, you will have to pay interest on the amount unpaid.

The Revenue has the right to make enquiries on tax returns, but it must normally let you know within 12 months of the filing deadline. The Revenue does not need a reason for choosing any particular return, and it will choose a few returns entirely at random.

Always put enough money on one side to pay your tax bills. I always keep a separate account for this. Provided you are not earning enough to put yourself in the highest tax band, put away about one quarter of what you earn. Your tax bill should not be as big as this, so you should have some extra money on one side for paying lump sum business expenses, such as your accountant, professional fees and perhaps some money to put towards capital expenses like a fax machine or mobile phone.

NATIONAL INSURANCE

In addition to income tax, you may also need to pay National Insurance contributions. As soon as you start doing locums, you should tell the local office of the Department of Social Security, even if you continue to work partly for an employer and partly for yourself. They will advise you on what your payments will be, how to pay them and they offer a range of leaflets covering the various levels of contributions.

Self-employed individuals normally have to pay Class 2 contributions at a flat weekly rate (£6.35 in 1998/9). If you expect your annual earnings to be below £3590, you can claim exemption from this liability. These contributions are collected by the Department of Social Security and you can pay them either by sticking stamps on a card or by direct debit.

In addition to Class 2 contributions, you will also have to pay Class 4 contributions on trading profits between certain limits. In 1998/9, the lower limit was £7310 and the upper limit was £25 220. The rate in 1998/9 was 6 per cent, but this does fluctuate a bit from year to year. Class 4 contributions are incorporated in the calculation of the balancing payment of income tax which is due on January 31 following the tax year.

Table 9.2   Worked example (1998/9 tax rates)

Let's say you are a single person and you work full time as a locum with no other earned income. Your locum earnings for the year were £25 000.

    Income = £25 000
    Personal allowance = £4195
    Business expenses and other tax allowances = £3000
    Taxable income = £25 000 − (£4195 + £3000)
                    = £17 805
Income tax = 20% of £4300 = £860
                23% of (£17 805 − £4300) = £3106.15
    Total income tax = £3996.15
National Insurance
    Class 2 = £6.35 per week = £330.20
    Class 4 = 6% of (£17 805 − £7310) = £629.70
    Total national insurance = £959.90
Total tax and national insurance = £4926.05

Table 9.2 shows a worked example of income tax liability and National Insurance contributions.

AN ACCOUNTANT

Good accountants should be able to save you the cost of their fees and more. If you work full time as a locum, or your tax affairs are complicated, it is probably worth considering having one. An accountant will be able to advise you on the best way to keep accounts and will provide information on allowable expenses, including those involved when you are starting out as a locum. But also check how much you can expect to pay your accountant for preparing your accounts and tax return.

PROTECTING YOUR SELF-EMPLOYED STATUS

The Inland Revenue has recently focused attention on locum pharmacists and has in some cases attempted to argue that locums are employees. This has implications for income tax and National Insurance contributions. In general, you are deemed to be employed rather than self employed, unless you have established a contract for services. You can do this by filling in a locum agreement form and keeping a copy of it (see Chapter 3). This represents minimum legal requirements to establish that there is a contract FOR service not a contract OF service; in the latter case you are deemed to be an employee.

The Inland Revenue and NI Contributions Agency will usually accept this agreement form as evidence of your self-employed status. You should also supply an invoice/receipt to the proprietor for your locum services and refer to the money you receive as fees rather than salary or wages. In addition, the Inland Revenue is less likely to query your self-employed status if your engagements are short (e.g. less than two months) and if you work for more than one owner or company.

However, the Inland Revenue reserves the right to question the actual practice of the parties concerned. The conditions of the contract must be observed or the legal position is open to challenge. As with any written agreement, it is of no consequence if its terms are not observed.

10

Insurance and pensions

Being self employed has many compensations, but remember that there is no-one to pay you a salary when you are sick and no company pension scheme. This means that you have to plan for your future and provide for such eventualities by considering insurance. The main types of insurance you might consider are:

○ Professional indemnity (see below).

○ Personal accident or sickness – cover against accidental death, permanent total disablement and temporary total disablement. If you have paid sufficient National Insurance contributions, you will be eligible for basic sickness benefit, but this is only a small weekly payment. You may want to take out sickness insurance on top of this. The Pharmaceutical and General Provident Society (Telephone: 01727 832161) offer a scheme for all pharmacists, including locums.

○ Life insurance.

○ Motor insurance – check your insurance policy to make sure you are covered for business.

○ Office equipment insurance – loss or damage to computer, fax machine etc. Check whether your home contents insurance already covers you for this.

PROFESSIONAL INDEMNITY

Wherever you work, you need to make sure that you are covered by professional indemnity insurance. With the diversification of pharmacists' duties and an increasingly litigation conscious general public, the risks of being taken to court are growing.

However, if you are working for a pharmacist or multiple who is in NPA membership, you are automatically covered by the member's professional indemnity insurance. NPA members are provided with a wide range of professional and third party insurance by the Chemists' Defence Association. This cover extends to claims arising from the activities of the NPA member plus any person employed or engaged in the pharmacy. This includes locums.

Always check the situation with regard to professional indemnity before accepting a booking. Ask if the pharmacy is in NPA membership, and make sure that the cover is in force. Phone the NPA if you are unsure; they will be quite happy to check this for you. Indeed, if you work for a pharmacy that is not an NPA member, you should enquire carefully about any cover that is in force and whether it extends to you. A proprietor's policy may have lapsed, the policy may cover the pharmacy and the owner but not a locum, and it is often difficult to get sight of the relevant documents.

If you want to accept work with pharmacies who are not in NPA membership, you should consider obtaining your own professional indemnity insurance. This will cost you about £150 a year.

Even if you are working exclusively for NPA members, what you might want to think about is cover against possible legal costs in the event of a prosecution. The Chemists' Defence Association covers members and any other person engaged in the member's business – this includes locums – against the costs of legal defence, provided that the alleged offence is not committed against the member and there is no conflict of interest between the member and the accused person.

If, for example, you as a locum unlawfully supplied a POM without a prescription or a P medicine was sold without your supervision, the NPA member could be prosecuted, but the alleged offence could be considered to have been committed against the member. You could then be prosecuted (possibly in addition to the proprietor) and in that event the Chemists' Defence Association would not cover the cost of your legal representation. The possibility of this happening is remote, but you may decide to insure yourself against the possibility of having to pay legal costs.

PENSIONS

If you are self employed, you should consider having a personal pension. But remember that there are a great number of pension schemes around, all of which will be extolled vigorously by pensions sales staff. It is best to seek advice on the choice of a pension scheme from a registered pensions broker.

The amount you can contribute to a personal pension plan depends on your age. Thus, if you are 35 or under, you can contribute 17.5 per cent of your income; as you get older, this percentage increases on a sliding scale. Investing in a pension scheme is not just a method of providing income when you eventually retire, it is also probably the most tax beneficial way of saving and investment. The main benefits are that:

O   You get tax relief on your contributions at your top rate of tax on earned income.

O   Your pension fund is itself tax exempt, so your capital builds up more rapidly than it would do in stocks and shares.

O   When you retire, you can have part of your benefits as a lump sum (which is not liable to capital gains tax) and part as a regular pension payment.

O   If you die, a lump sum is paid to your dependents free of inheritance tax.

O   Your pension is portable and remains your property, even if you subsequently join a company with its own pension scheme.

Appendix 1

REFERENCE SOURCES

British National Formulary. London: The British Medical Association and the Royal Pharmaceutical Society of Great Britain. (Published twice a year. All pharmacies will have a copy of this, but you may prefer to buy your own.)

Medicines, Ethics and Practice: A guide for pharmacists. London: The Royal Pharmaceutical Society of Great Britain. (Published twice a year.)

OTC Directory. Treatments for Common Ailments. London: Proprietary Association of Great Britain. (Published yearly. Many pharmacies have a copy of this.)

Chemist & Druggist. Guide to OTC Medicines. (Published twice a year. All pharmacies who subscribe to the *Chemist & Druggist* will have a copy of this.)

FURTHER READING

Blenkinsopp A, Paxton P (1998) *Symptoms in the Pharmacy: A guide to the management of common illness.* 3rd edition. Oxford: Blackwell Science. This book provides guidance on responding to symptoms in community pharmacy. It covers areas of questioning, referral to general practitioners and choice of treatment.

Edwards C, Stillman P (1995) *Minor Illness or Major Disease? Responding to symptoms in the pharmacy.* 2nd edition. London: Pharmaceutical Press. This book describes a rational approach to distinguishing between patients' symptoms which can be managed by a pharmacist and those which need referral to a general practitioner. Selection of appropriate over-the-counter medicines for each condition is also covered.

Harman R (1989) *Patient Care in Community Practice: A handbook of non-medicinal health-care*. London: Pharmaceutical Press. This book is a guide to a range of products and appliances (e.g. stoma appliances, incontinence aids, oxygen therapy, special dietary products, graduated compression hosiery and inhalation therapy aids) used in the community.

Li Wan Po A, Li Wan Po G (1997) *OTC Medications: Symptoms and treatment of common illnesses*. 2nd edition. Oxford: Blackwell Science. This book provides a reference of common ailments and the OTC medicines which can be used to treat them.

Nathan A (1998) *Non-prescription Medicines*. London: Pharmaceutical Press. This book provides a reference of common ailments and the OTC medicines which can be used to treat them.

Appendix 2

The Royal Pharmaceutical
Society of Great Britain
1 Lambeth High Street
London SE1 7JN
Tel: 0171 735 9141
Fax: 0171 735 7629

The National
Pharmaceutical Association
Mallinson House
38–42 St Peter's Street
St Albans
Hertfordshire AL1 3NP
Tel: 01727 832161
Fax: 01727 840858

Pharmaceutical Services
Negotiating Committee
59 Buckingham Street
Aylesbury
Buckinghamshire HP20 2PJ
Tel: 01296 432823
Fax: 01296 392181

Centre for Pharmacy Post-
graduate Education (CPPE)
Pharmacy Department

University of Manchester
Oxford Road
Manchester M13 9PL
Tel: 0161 275 2324
Fax: 0161 275 2419

Scottish Centre for
Pharmacy Postgraduate
Education (SCPPE)
University of Strathclyde
204 George Street
Glasgow G1 1XW
Tel: 0141 552 4400
Fax: 0141 552 6443

Welsh Centre for
Postgraduate
Pharmaceutical Education
(WCPPE)
Welsh School of Pharmacy
Cardiff University
King Edward VII Avenue
Cathays Park
Cardiff CF1 3XF
Tel: 01222 874782
Fax: 01222 874149

LOCUM AGENCIES

Apotek Locums
95–97 Melton Road
Leicester LE4 6PN
Tel: 0116 268 2174
Fax: 0116 268 2174

Capital Locums
93–99 George Lane
South Woodford
London E18 1AN
Tel: 0181 532 9980
Fax: 0181 532 9980

Direct Locums
23 St Ann's Park Road
Wandsworth
London SW18 2RW
Tel: 0973 755556
Fax: 0181 875 0707

Elite Recruitment Specialists
20 Grosvenor Place
Belgravia
London SW1X 7HN
Tel: 0171 235 1900
Fax: 0171 235 4615

Essential Locum Services Ltd
11 Abbotts Road
Kings Heath
Birmingham
West Midlands B14 7QD

Tel: 0121 444 0075
Fax: 0121 444 0084

Jenrick Medical Ltd
145–147 Frimley Road
Camberley
Surrey GU15 2PS
Tel: 01276 676141
Fax: 01276 676050

JPM Group
Marshal House
22 Fontayne Avenue
Chigwell
Essex IG7 5HF
Tel: 0181 502 6349
Fax: 0181 502 6361

The Locum Agency
20 Perth Avenue
Kings Park
Bradford BD2 1EE
Tel: 01274 720884
Fax: 01274 731917

Locum Link
Brent House
214 Kenton Road
Kenton
Middlesex HA3 8DJ
Tel: 0181 907 9894
Fax: 0181 909 1041

Frank G May & Son
3 St Michael's Road
Maidstone
Kent ME16 8BS
Tel: 01622 754427
Fax: 01622 754427

Medic International
1st Floor
25 King Street
Twickenham TW1 3SD
Tel: 0181 744 3035
Fax: 0181 892 6564

MEDACS
6 Paddington Street
London W1M 4BE
Tel:0171 935 1506
Fax: 0171 224 4924

Meka Locums
Merlin House
122–126 Kilburn High Road
London NW6 4HY
Tel: 0171 372 3399
Fax: 0171 624 8202

Northern Locums
13 Winchester Road
Radcliffe
Manchester M26 0LY
Tel: 0161 725 8063

Pharm-Assist
Wharfe Bank Cottage

Ings Road
Ulleskelf
Tadcaster LF24 9SS
Tel: 01937 833300
Fax: 01937 833644

Principal Locums
Morgan House
249 Cranbrook Road
Ilford
Essex IG1 4TG
Tel: 0181 252 5471
Fax: 0181 252 5277

Provincial Pharmacy Locum Services
The Old Fire Station
69 Albion Street
Birmingham B1 3EA
Tel: 0121 233 0233
Fax: 0121 693 0038

R & G Locums
11 Stockbridge Road
Donagadhee
County Down BT21 0PN
Tel: 01247 883034
Fax: 01247 883034

Judi Wilson Associates
1 Hailes Park
Edinburgh EH13 0NG
Tel: 0131 441 4445
Fax: 0131 467 7476

Index